THE PROSTATE CANCER ESSENTIALS FOR SURVIVAL SERIES

HORMONAL THERAPY FOR PROSTATE CANCER: THE BENEFITS AND RISKS

MICHAEL J. DATTOLI, MD

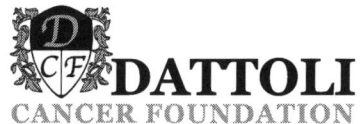

SARASOTA, FLORIDA

Hormonal Therapy for Prostate Cancer

Copyright © 2017 by Michael J. Dattoli, M.D.

All rights reserved. No part of this work may be reproduced or transmitted in any form or by any means, electronic or mechanical, including photocopying or recording, or by any information storage or retrieval system, except as may be expressly permitted by the 1976 Copyright Act or in writing by the publisher.

ISBN-10: 1-5429102-6-9
ISBN-13: 978-1-5429-1026-2

Published by the Dattoli Cancer Foundation, Sarasota, FL
Imprint of record: CreateSpace, Charleston, SC
Book design and composition by Dan van Loon, Batavia, IL

MEDICAL DISCLAIMER

This book is intended as a supplement but not as a substitute for the medical advice of a physician. It is imperative that you consult a qualified healthcare professional with regard to all matters relating to your health and particular situation. Neither the publisher nor the authors bear responsibility for any consequences due to the reader's decision to use any particular treatment, medication, dietary supplement or other healthcare practices discussed in this book.

DEDICATION

This book is dedicated to all those whose lives have been touched by prostate cancer, and to the patients and their families whom we are privileged to serve and educate as cancer care providers.

ACKNOWLEDGMENTS

We are deeply grateful to a number of people who have contributed to this booklet. Our thanks to Greg Lawrence, for his editorial efforts and to Ginya Carnahan, Chris Wells, Jone Fay, Meg Brockett, and Jennifer Hogan, MLT, ASCP, at the Dattoli Cancer Center & Brachytherapy Research Institute for their ongoing assistance.

We also want to thank Jennifer Cash ARNP, MS, for her long association and many contributions to the Dattoli Cancer Foundation and this booklet series. We deeply appreciate all of those wonderful patients and family members who have contacted the Dattoli Cancer Foundation for counseling and guidance and in turn have given us their support and encouragement. It is your spirit and commitment in confronting this disease that inspires us all.

CONTENTS

INTRODUCTION

A Personal Choice: Hormonal Therapy 9

OVERVIEW—HORMONAL THERAPY

What is Hormonal Therapy and How Does It Work? 11
How Does Hormonal Therapy Kill Cancer Cells? 13
What is Orchiectomy? 13
What is Estrogen Therapy? 14
What is LHRH Therapy? 15
What is Combined Hormonal Therapy? 16
What is Triple Hormonal Therapy? 17
What is Intermittent Hormonal Therapy? 18
How are Patients Monitored with Hormonal Therapy? 18
What Determines How Long Hormonal Therapy is Effective? 18
When Should Hormonal Therapy be Initiated? 19
What Options are Available Once Hormonal Therapy Stops Working? 21
What is Neoadjuvant Hormonal Therapy? 21
Potential Side Effects of Androgen Deprivation Therapy 22
What are the Pros and Cons of the Various Hormonal Therapies? 24
Hormonal Therapy, DART and Brachytherapy 26

APPENDICES

A: Deciding What is Best for You 29
B: Glossary of Medical Terms 31
C: The Warning Signs of Prostate Cancer 45

About the Author 46
The Dattoli Cancer Foundation Mission 47
Order More Booklets in the Series 48

INTRODUCTION

A PERSONAL CHOICE: HORMONAL THERAPY

Having spent more than twenty five years studying prostate cancer and treating thousands of men, I am well aware that this is one of the most controversial fields of medicine. This is especially true with regard to hormonal therapy (also known as *androgen deprivation therapy, or ADT*). Because there is considerable disagreement among doctors about the use of hormones, it is advisable for each patient to discuss this treatment option carefully with his physician. If you are a patient and have uncertainties about whether hormonal therapy is appropriate in your case, it would be wise to obtain a second opinion. Patients are also advised to contact support groups and talk with other patients who have undergone one or more of the various forms of ADT.

Hormonal therapy is not appropriate for every patient, and we have written this booklet to answer the most common questions about hormones, and to help you decide if this therapy may be right for you. Before deciding on any form of treatment, you should fully investigate the likelihood of cure and the risk of side effects that may alter your quality of life. These are the most important considerations in deciding on treatment. Given your age, overall health, and the stage of the cancer, you will want to find a balance between treatment effectiveness and side effects—a balance with which you are comfortable, that you can live with both before and after treatment. Knowing what to expect each step of the way is one of the keys to fighting this disease.

This booklet will explain the pros and cons of hormonal therapy, as a *primary therapy* for patients with advanced disease and for older patients who are unable to tolerate other therapies. We will also discuss ADT as a *secondary therapy* used in conjunction with curative or salvage therapies such as advanced radiotherapy and surgery. Patients need to become informed about hormones in order to weigh the benefits and the risks in each individual case.

—Michael J. Dattoli, M.D.

OVERVIEW

HORMONAL THERAPY

While hormonal therapy is controversial, no one disputes the fact that this form of treatment has benefited many patients. It should be stressed, however, that hormonal therapy is not considered a cure for prostate cancer. Some patients on hormones fare better than others over time. Hormonal therapy is used in various ways either as a monotherapy or in conjunction with other forms of therapy.

The discussion of hormones often becomes very technical, but the effort to wade through this material may help you to understand how hormonal therapy works and to make an informed judgment as to whether or not this form of therapy may be beneficial for you.

What is Hormonal Therapy and How Does It Work?

In 1941, Charles Huggins M.D. and Clarence Hodges M.D. reported that androgen deprivation was an effective aid for advanced prostate cancer patients, a discovery that led to a Nobel Prize in 1966. Hormonal therapy has since become a standard palliative treatment for those patients whose cancer has spread beyond the prostate gland. At present, nothing works better for advanced prostate cancer than hormonal therapy, also known as Androgen Deprivation Therapy (ADT) in its various forms. If after radiation therapy or surgery or cryosurgery, there is evidence of a rising PSA (biochemical failure) or a positive biopsy, hormonal therapy is likely to be considered along with other salvage therapies.

Increasingly, men with less advanced prostate cancer are also opting for hormonal therapy, either alone or in combination with radiation or surgery. When hormonal intervention is used to downsize the tumor prior to a primary treatment, it is referred to as *neoadjuvant* therapy. Some men elect to undergo hormonal therapy instead of a primary therapy (radiation, surgery, or cryosurgery) because of individual health considerations, advanced age, fear of side effects, and so forth.

Hormonal therapy takes a variety of forms, both surgical (orchiectomy, though much less common these days for reasons explained below) and chemical or medical ADT, all of which rely on a common strategy for attacking the cancer by reducing levels of circulating testosterone. It has long been known that prostate cancer is to some extent dependent on and nourished by the male sex hormone, testosterone. This is one of a group of hormones known as *androgens*.

The androgens are responsible for the masculine body changes associated with puberty: growth of body hair, increased muscle mass and genital size, and the deepening of a man's voice. Testosterone also regulates sexual desire, and influences moods and aggressiveness. Like other hormones, testosterone is a chemical released in the body through various biochemical mechanisms and carried in the bloodstream, where it can be detected by a blood test.

Since testosterone stimulates the growth of prostate cancer cells, depleting or ablating the body's testosterone tends to shrink the size of many tumors, specifically, those that are hormone-sensitive. The goal of hormonal therapy is to decrease the production of testosterone in the body, inhibiting the growth and progression of the cancer. These hormone-sensitive prostate cancers essentially are put into remission by the removal of the body's testosterone. In most cases, hormonal therapy will also significantly reduce pain and other symptoms of the disease when it has metastasized. Because hormonal therapy works against the body's production of the male hormones, it might be more accurately described as "anti-hormonal therapy."

Erectile dysfunction and loss of sexual desire are likely with almost every form of hormonal therapy. At least 95% of patients lose sexual desire and the ability to have an erection. Some of the newer hormonal agents discussed below have shown improvement in maintaining sexual function.

While as many as 85% of prostate cancers are responsive to hormonal ablation, individual patient response to hormonal therapy varies widely. For those who initially respond to treatment, control of the disease may last from several months to many years. Two years is the average. As many as 10% of patients with metastatic disease survive for ten years or more, while more than 25% are still alive after five years. 80% of patients experience some relief of pain. However, in most cases, the cancer eventually becomes resistant to treatment, or *refractory*, and the patient will experience a relapse of the disease. This occurs because some of the cancer cells mutate and become *androgen-independent,* meaning that they are unaffected by male hormones. At this point, no form of hormonal therapy is likely to have a significant impact on the disease. Patients with androgen-independent prostate cancer

(AIPC) can still utilize other forms of treatment, such as a second line of androgen ablation therapy followed by chemotherapy and various chemical agents, which are often administered through clinical trials (see "What Options are Available Once Hormonal Therapy Stops Working?").

In our practice we utilize a variety of regimes which may slow or stop prostate cancer growth, with chemotherapy considered as a last resort. These regimens for patients with advanced disease may include agents such as Casodex®, Avodart®, estrogenic agents, Thalidomide, Cox-II inhibitors, agents which disrupt the IGF-1 pathway, Ketoconazole, and agents to improve bone integrity (bisphosphonate), which not only counteract the adverse effects of hormones on bones, but which are also antineoplastic (having anti-cancer effects). Some of these agents are described in greater detail. We also prescribe hormones in conjunction with radiotherapy, in order to enhance the cancer-killing efficacy of radiation. Because of potentially serious side effects with ADT, in our practice, we usually limit hormones to 12 to 13 months or less. We also prescribe medications to lessen side effects in the short term, as discussed in greater depth below.

How Does Hormonal Therapy Kill Cancer Cells?

Androgen deprivation causes what is known as programmed cell death, or *apoptosis*, which affects those cancer cells that are hormone-dependent. This results from a biochemical process referred to as *enzymatic DNA degradation*. Enzymes (often called "suicide enzymes") within the cell break down the genetic memory code and cause the cell to die. The mechanism of programmed cell death caused by androgen deprivation involves a long, complicated chain of biochemical events within each cell. Exactly how this process takes place is under continuing study by researchers who are seeking to develop more effective chemical agents to treat the disease. The challenge is to develop agents that kill the cancer cells without harming healthy prostate cells.

What is an Orchiectomy?

A bilateral orchiectomy involves the surgical removal of the testicles from the scrotal sack. This procedure is also known as surgical castration. Orchiectomy is one of several hormonal options for patients with late stage prostate cancer, though for most patients, this surgical procedure is the least appealing and is only rarely performed these days. Most men are prescribed injectable hormonal agents instead. Surgical castration provides a baseline for comparison with other forms of ADT.

The testicles produce about 95 percent of the body's testosterone, and after their removal, a dramatic impact is often observed on prostate cancer, with a marked fall in the serum PSA level. Orchiectomy usually results in a retardation of the growth and spread of the cancer. Most tumors (both primary and metastatic) shrink in size after a bilateral orchiectomy is performed. Patients also experience a significant alleviation of pain and other symptoms. In most cases, the benefits of orchiectomy will be temporary, and eventually the disease will reassert itself. Nevertheless, the procedure has been shown to stave off the symptomatic effects of the disease for many months or years, as do other nonsurgical forms of ADT.

Although the operation is minor and can be performed on an out-patient basis, using general or local anesthesia, most men find this surgery difficult to accept, even those patients who are no longer sexually active. The side effects associated with castrate testosterone levels vary considerably from patient to patient. Most men will experience loss of sexual desire and impotence following a bilateral orchiectomy. Hot flashes are a common side effect of the operation, affecting about one third of patients. Hot flashes involve a sudden rush of heat to the face, neck, upper chest, and back, lasting from a few seconds to an hour. These symptoms can be counteracted or ameliorated by various medications.

Orchiectomy may also cause mood changes, such as irritability or a loss of aggressiveness. Loss of muscle mass, weight gain, bone loss (osteopenia and osteoporosis) and changes in skin tone and hair growth are often late effects of treatment. Compared to other forms of hormonal therapy, a major disadvantage of bilateral orchiectomy is that it is irreversible.

What is Estrogen Therapy?

The administration of the female hormone, estrogen, inhibits the production of testosterone. Until recent years, this was the most common form of androgen deprivation therapy. When the pituitary gland in the brain detects the presence of female hormones, it stops production of male hormones by the testicles. Estrogenic compounds block the signal transmitted by the pituitary gland, known as luteinizing hormone (LH), which normally stimulates testosterone production. In the past, the most commonly prescribed form of estrogen was diethylstilbestrol, or DES®, taken orally. DES® is cheaper than most other hormone medications, but is no longer commonly prescribed because of the risk of blood clots. However, this risk is effectively countered by using blood thinners such as Coumadin. Estrogens have for the most part been replaced by LHRH agonists and anti-androgens, although estrogens remain an option when LHRH agonists and anti-androgens cease to work (see "What is LHRH therapy?").

Studies have shown DES® and other estrogenic agents, such as estradiol, to be as effective as orchiectomy for temporarily halting the progression of prostate cancer. However, like orchiectomy, there are a number of side effects associated with estrogen therapy. These include fluid retention, breast enlargement and tenderness (gynecomastia), loss of sexual desire and erectile dysfunction, and rarely nausea and vomiting. Even more serious, estrogen therapy may result in severe circulatory or thrombotic problems, such as blood clots and stroke. Estradiol patches can eliminate the risk of life-threatening thrombotic events that are associated with other hormonal agents. .

Aside from DES® and estradiol, other drugs that have been used for estrogen therapy include Premarin® and ethinyl estradiol, which are medications also used by some women during menopause. These also include Evamist® spray, Divigel, and Minivelle® patches. Transdermal patches such as Estraderm® and Vivelle-Dot®, and Climara® are used to avoid metabolism of estrogen within the liver, and thereby reduce the risk of dangerous thrombotic side effects. Polyestradiol intramuscular (Estradurin®) may also be prescribed, administered by monthly injection. Another estrogen drug sometimes prescribed is estramustine phosphate (EMCYT®), which is taken orally, but it too carries the risk of serious side effects.

What is LHRH Therapy?

This form of hormonal therapy utilizes *leutinizing hormone releasing hormone* (LHRH) agonists (or analogs), a synthesized form of a natural brain hormone. LHRH agonists effectively shut down production of testicular testosterone, achieving the same effect as surgical removal of the testicles, however, the effects are not permanent. This type of hormonal therapy is sometimes referred to as chemical castration, or medical castration.

LHRH agonists currently available in the U.S. include leuprolide (Lupron®, Viadur®, and Eligard®), goserelin (Zoladex®), and triptorelin (TRELSTAR®). LHRH agonists may be injected monthly or every 3, 4, or 12 months in the physician's office. Degarelix (trade name Firmagon®) is an LHRH antagonist. It works like the LHRH agonists, but it lowers testosterone levels more quickly and doesn't cause tumor flare like the LHRH agonists do, as discussed below.

LHRH therapy has been a great benefit to those men who wish to avoid surgery. However, LHRH therapy is not without its disadvantages. The drugs are expensive, as they can cost $350 or more per month, which may be prohibitively high for some patients, although most insurance companies cover the cost in full (Medicare included). The side effects of LHRH agonists are similar to those associated with bilateral orchiectomy, namely hot flashes, some loss of libido, weight-gain, and in some cases erectile dysfuncton. Infrequent gastrointestinal side effects have been reported as well. The LHRH agonists are usually used in conjunction with other oral agents rather than as a monotherapy.

What is Combined Hormonal Therapy?

A "flare reaction" is observed when LHRH therapy is initiated, causing a brief rise or surge in testosterone level. The testosterone flare is accompanied by a rise in PSA and subsequent increase of cancer symptoms, such as bone pain and urinary difficulties in some men. This initial phase typically lasts only a week or two. Small doses of estrogenic compounds, or *anti-androgens* such as bicalutamide (Casodex®), nilutamide (Nilandron®), and cyproterone acetate (Androcur®) may be administered 7 days prior to the initiation of LHRH therapy, as they act to block this flare phenomenon. The anti-androgens block the effects of rising testosterone levels without impacting estrogen levels. This is a form of combined hormonal therapy, utilizing more than one hormonal agent. The anti-androgens prevent attachment of testosterone to prostate cells, and they are used to block the small percentage of testosterone produced by the adrenal glands.

The testosterone surge caused by LHRH therapy can be detrimental, as it may promote cancer growth and potential dissemination. Unfortunately, all too many patients having localized prostate cancer receive LHRH agonists by their urologists without being given opposing agents such as estrogenic compounds or anti-androgens. This is an area of treatment about which urologists are often not as informed as oncologists, and may do more harm than good.

The anti-androgen drugs may also cause side effects such as breast enlargement and nipple tenderness. These problems can be avoided by a short course of radiation therapy administered to the breast tissue. About 10% of men experience nausea and/or diarrhea when taking anti-androgens. There is also some small risk of liver damage, and therefore, a blood test to check liver enzymes is usually given every three months.

Abarelix (trade name Plenaxis) is an LHRH antagonist like Degarelix (Firmagon®) that has been shown to induce castration-level testosterone without the temporary testosterone surge associated with drugs like Lupron®, Zoladex®, TRELSTAR®, and Viadur®. Often prescribed for patients with bone metastases, Abarelix also reduces pain and urinary symptoms. However, a small percentage of men (less than 5%) have serious allergic reactions to the drug. Abarelix is administered by injection every 2 weeks for the first month, and every 4 weeks thereafter. Patients are monitored for a half hour after being injected to be sure they do not show signs of allergic reaction.

What is Triple Hormonal Therapy?

This form of treatment combines the use of LHRH agonists with an anti-androgen, and *5-alpha reductase inhibitor,* usually finasteride (Proscar®) or dutasteride (Avodart®). In the prostate gland, 5-alpha reductase is an enzyme that converts testosterone into a more potent growth stimulator or metabolite, dihydrotestosterone (DHT). This enzyme is blocked by the 5-alpha reductase inhibitors such as Proscar®, thus inhibiting the production of DHT. Many researchers now believe that the 5-alpha reductase inhibitors improve the efficacy of hormonal therapy.

A National Cancer Institute study demonstrated that Proscar® actually prevents cancer for 25% of those patients taking the drug. That same study also reported that Proscar® encouraged more aggressive cancers in a small percentage of men, but that finding has since been refuted. It appears that tissue biopsies of those receiving Proscar® were falsely interpreted as being more aggressive.

Other recent studies have indicated that combination triple hormonal blockade is superior to other forms of hormonal therapy, extending the average period of remission by several months. In addition, the percentage of patients who respond to therapy is higher, and more men experience complete remission. However, clinical evaluation has been somewhat contradictory concerning the advantages of combination therapy over monotherapy (the use of a single hormonal regimen to suppress androgen production).

A modified combination therapy that uses Casodex® with finasteride (Proscar® or Avodart®) allows many men to preserve potency while undergoing hormonal therapy. This limited combination of hormones (often referred to as Sequential Androgen Blockade, or SAB) can preserve quality of life, as neither of these drugs impact on sexual function to the extent that other hormonal agents do.

The mechanism of the SAB combination acts to block testosterone (and its more potent metabolite, DHT) on the cellular level of the tumor, while maintaining normal testosterone levels in the bloodstream, with the hope that the patient's sexual function will be preserved. However, with this approach there is a risk of breast enlargement and hypersensitivity of the nipples. These side effects can be counteracted by a short course of radiation delivered to the breast before starting therapy, or by administering drugs such as anastrozole (Arimidex®) to relieve the symptoms after they appear. Another approach using Casodex® at three times the typical daily dose (150 mg daily) achieves similar results without the dramatic impact on bone integrity and sexual dysfunction.

What is Intermittent Hormonal Therapy?

Intermittent hormonal therapy is a technique that offers the advantage of sparing patients side effects during intervals when they go off therapy. As previously noted, nearly all prostate cancers treated with androgen deprivation therapy become resistant to this treatment over a period of months or years. Many researchers believe that constant androgen suppression may not be necessary, so they recommend intermittent (on-again, off-again) therapy.

At our institution, utilizing this approach, combination hormonal therapy (an LHRH agonist and an anti-androgen, plus or minus Proscar® or Avodart®) may be used for at least six months or more, and then stopped once the patient's PSA drops to an undetectable level. If the PSA level begins to rise to a predetermined value (e.g. 5 to 10), the drugs are started again. The off-phase of therapy can range from several months to several years or more, during which time many patients can recover sexual potency and quality of life. The resumption of the body's production of testosterone eventually restores normal blood testosterone levels and resolves most side effects caused by hormonal therapy; however, recovery time varies, and some patients are slower than others to recover their natural testosterone production.

How are Patients Monitored with Hormonal Therapy?

Patients are typically monitored every six months with a digital rectal exam, a PSA test, and chemistries to test for kidney function and liver function. Testosterone levels are tested every 4 to 6 weeks while patients are on ADT. If the PSA begins to rise, patients are given a bone scan once or twice a year to test for bone metastases. A blood test will also be used to measure the level of testosterone, to be sure it is within the castrate range and not fluctuating. With anti-androgens such as Casodex®, a blood test for liver enzymes is usually performed every 6 to 8 weeks and then every three months if stable. In addition, a number of medications are commonly prescribed to ensure bone integrity, in which case, calcium and magnesium levels require monitoring.

What Determines How Long Hormonal Therapy is Effective after Other Treatments have been Exhausted??

The benefits of hormonal therapy vary considerably from patient to patient when used as a monotherapy after radiation, surgery and other primary treatments that have not been effective in eradicating the cancer.

It is often reported that hormonal therapy is effective for an average of 18 months, but the length of time varies considerably and some patients continue to respond to ADT for many years.

Two factors appear to determine how long hormonal therapy is effective: the number of hormone-sensitive cells compared to the number of hormone-independent cells, and how fast the cancer is growing (the rate at which the cancer doubles in size). It is the hormone-independent cells that are ultimately fatal, and therefore, the rate at which they are growing is crucial. Research in the field is now focused on controlling these hormone-resistant cancer cells. If you are just beginning hormonal therapy today, it is entirely possible that new treatments will be available by the time hormones have ceased to work for you.

When Should Hormonal Therapy be Initiated?

During recent years there has been a growing enthusiasm for the early initiation of hormonal therapy, especially combination hormonal therapy. Early initiation means starting hormonal therapy before any symptoms of metastatic disease appear. Advocates of this approach point to those studies that indicate some degree of local control achieved with hormonal agents, slowing progression of the disease. It might appear to be common sense that because hormonal therapy lowers PSA, shrinks tumors and slows progression of the cancer, that it would also prolong life. But this may not be the case. Although the benefits of hormonal therapy for treating prostate cancer have been established, there is considerable controversy about how effective hormonal therapy may be at increasing survival.

Researchers remain divided on the optimal time to begin therapy, though recent studies favor early versus late initiation of hormonal therapy. The argument against early use of hormones rests on the fact that those who opt for early initiation will not be able to use hormonal therapy later when symptoms appear. By that time, the tumor may have become androgen-independent and refractory. After the beneficial effects of hormonal therapy have run their course, a patient's cancer may begin to grow again and eventually progress to what it would have been had hormonal therapy never been given. With this in mind, some doctors encourage men with advanced disease to embark on a course of active surveillance, arguing that these patients should avoid side effects as long as possible since the treatment has not been shown to substantially prolong life. This conservative strategy calls for the use of hormone therapy only if and when symptoms appear.

Other researchers argue that men with metastatic disease yet smaller tumors and low Gleason scores (less aggressive cancer) might even be cured if treatment is started sooner because these patients have less cancer to begin with and slower growing cancer. As a tumor grows and becomes bulky, genetic changes may take place within the cancer cells that lead to androgen-independence; therefore, early treatment might offer some advantage for these patients by attacking the cancer before it becomes refractory. This point of view is supported by a Mayo Clinic non-randomized study which indicated that patients with positive lymph nodes and low Gleason scores lived longer if they were treated hormonally before symptoms appeared.

Early initiation of hormonal therapy may indeed halt disease progression temporarily while these patients evaluate other primary treatment options. But a number of studies have demonstrated that early hormonal intervention prior to radical surgery does not reduce the risk of biochemical failure. However, the early use of hormones appears to be more advantageous before undertaking radiation as a primary therapy. Our own patients who received hormones had very aggressive tumors, and yet they fared similarly to those low risk patients who did not receive hormones. As the high risk group would have been expected to fare much worse, this would therefore support the use of hormones in this group. In addition, numerous multi-institutional studies both in the U.S. and abroad have demonstrated a benefit with the utilization of hormonal therapy prior to, during and after radiation (see the RTOG clinical trials cited below).

It is clear that more men regardless of the stage of their cancer are choosing to initiate hormonal therapy early because of a perceived possibility of cure, or long-term remission. This option may seem appealing given the steady progress in the field and the likely development of new and more effective chemical agents in the near future. However, before making this choice, patients should fully investigate the potential side effects and changes in quality of life that can be anticipated with hormonal manipulation. Men who opt for early combination hormonal therapy should also keep in mind that the hormones are likely to stop working eventually. Regardless of the stage of cancer, patients should also consider lifestyle changes, including diet and nutrition, and utilizing agents like Celebrex® and Zyflamend®.

Hormonal therapy continues to be controversial because there are still so many unanswered questions in this area, and because doctors disagree about what the answers will turn out to be. The nature of this controversy makes it all the more important for patients to question their doctors carefully before embarking on treatment. Be sure your doctor has considerable experience with hormonal therapy, and find out what that experience has been with other patients of similar age and stage of cancer as your own.

You should carefully discuss the pros and cons of each drug with your doctors and if you remain in doubt, by all means, obtain a second opinion. While the lack of definitive knowledge about hormonal therapy may be unsettling, each patient can still make an educated decision based on the possible benefits and risks associated with this form of treatment.

What Options are Available Once Hormonal Therapy Stops Working?

All combinations of hormonal therapy should be completely exhausted before further options are considered. For example, if the anti-androgen Casodex® ceases to be effective, as indicated by a rising PSA, consideration might be given to changing to another anti-androgen such as Nilandron® or Androcur®. There are a number of hormonal options available and new ones constantly being developed for FDA approval.

After patients with advanced disease have exhausted all of these hormonal measures, alternative options may include chemotherapy and clinical trials that offer experimental treatments such as immunotherapy and vaccine therapies. When the cancer becomes resistant to castration, docetaxel-based chemotherapy is the regulatory-approved standard of care, regardless of the patient's age. Cabazitaxel (Jevtana®) and abiraterone acetate (Zytiga®) have also been shown to prolong survival, irrespective of age, and are now in clinical use having received FDA approval, as have Provenge and Xtandi®. Further advances are being investigated, with promising results reported from phase III clinical trials.

What Is Neoadjuvant Hormonal Therapy?

Neoadjuvant Hormonal Therapy employs hormonal agents *before* primary curative therapies such as radical surgery (prostatectomy), radiation therapy, and cryosurgery. The primary goal of neoadjuvant therapy is to enhance the effectiveness of the primary therapy by shrinking the tumor before treatment. Some studies have suggested that positive surgical margins (cancer cells detected at the point of surgical resection during or following prostatectomy) may be reduced if the procedure is preceded by hormonal therapy. However, biochemical testing and biopsy five years following hormonal therapy and surgery have shown no improvement in freedom from failure (PSA recurrence), indicating that the outcome is not improved for patients with localized prostate cancer.

By contrast, a number of studies have shown improved results at local control of the disease and survival for higher risk patients when hormonal therapy is administered prior to and following external beam radiation therapy and brachytherapy. The landmark study in this area was a European clinical trial, EORTC 22863 (Eur Urol. 1998 Dec; 35 Suppl S1:23-26.). That was the first study to demonstrate an overall survival benefit of radiation therapy combined with hormones versus radiation alone.

Another clinical trial, RTOG 9202, published by the Radiation Therapy Oncology Group, showed that adjuvant ADT before, during and 24 months after RT showed a significant survival advantage for patients with Gleason scores 8 to 10 (Hanks et al, J Clin Oncol. 2003 Nov 1;21(21):3972-8). The dose of radiation utilized in these early clinical trials were low compared to our current dosimetry protocols with DART and brachytherapy.

Though not definitive, the results of these studies and others are seen as encouraging by many researchers. Many of us believe that hormonal therapy and radiation have a synergistic effect in eradicating the cancer, especially in high risk patients. At the same time, it should be noted that no advantage has been found for neoadjuvant ADT given with radiation for low-risk patients.

Recent studies of combined treatment modalities have also helped to determine our clinical protocol for combining ADT with brachytherapy, Dynamic Adaptive Radiation Therapy (DART), and all modalities associated with 4-Dimensional Image Guided Intensity Modulated Radiation Therapy (4D IG-IMRT). For additional information and guidance with regard to brachytherapy, DART and IMRT, readers are referred to our companion Prostate Cancer Essentials booklet, *IMRT with DART and Brachytherapy.*

Potential Side Effects of Androgen Deprivation Therapy

Like orchiectomy, LHRH agonists and antagonists can cause similar side effects from lower levels of androgens in the body. These side effects include:

- Diminished sexual desire
- Erectile dysfunction (impotence)
- Shrinkage of the testicles and penis
- Hot flashes
- Breast enlargement and tenderness
- Osteoporosis (loss of bone integrity)
- Anemia (low red blood cell counts)
- Impaired cognitive function (including memory loss, Alzheimer's disease and dementia)
- Loss of muscle mass
- Weight gain
- Fatigue

- Increased cholesterol levels
- Depression

Anti-androgens have a similar side effects profile; however, the major difference from LHRH agonists, antagonists and orchiectomy is that anti-androgens appear to have fewer sexual side effects. When the anti-androgen drugs are used alone, sexual desire and erectile functions can often be maintained. When anti-androgen drugs are given to patients who are also being treated with LHRH agonists, diarrhea is a major side effect. Nausea, fatigue and liver toxicity can also occur.

It should be noted that many side effects of hormone therapy can be prevented or ameliorated, including the following:

- Hot flashes can often be mitigated by treatment with various medications.
- Brief radiation treatment to the breasts can help prevent their enlargement, but this is not effective after breast enlargement has manifested.
- Several medications can help prevent and treat osteoporosis.
- Depression can be treated with antidepressant medications and/or counseling.
- Exercise and nutrition can help reduce or mitigate some side effects, such as fatigue, weight gain, and the loss of bone and muscle mass.

A number of recent studies have suggested that ADT also carries a significant risk of high blood pressure, diabetes, strokes, heart attacks and death from heart disease. Patients considering ADT should be aware that the likelihood of these more serious side effects with hormones increases over time while patients are undergoing ADT. For example, there is a significantly higher risk of cognitive impairment such as Alzheimer's disease and dementia after a year of hormonal therapy (Nead KT, et al, Association Between Androgen Deprivation Therapy and Risk of Dementia; JAMA Oncol. 2017 Jan 1;3(1):49-55). In our practice, in light of the dangers of comorbidities, we favor a very conservative approach and limit adjuvant hormonal therapy to 12 to 13 months or less. We encourage our patients to weigh the benefits and risks of ADT in light of age, overall health, and the specifics of each individual case.

While studies have shown that there is a risk of serious side effects that can lead to mortality with long-term use of ADT, those deaths have not been taken into account in the many studies of prostate cancer survival after treatment. Mortality due to the side effects of ADT is usually misrepresented in the data as deaths from causes other than prostate cancer; when in fact this type of mortality is being caused by the use of hormones to treat the disease. This means that there are actually more annual deaths from prostate cancer than reported.

What are the Pros and Cons of the Various Hormonal Therapies?

Orchiectomy

Pros
1. Easy, quick, effective surgery
2. No ongoing drug therapy
3. Relatively inexpensive compared to drugs

Cons
1. Psychological impact of castration
2. Does not supress adrenal androgens
3. Side effects including impotence, loss of libido, hot flashes
4. Irreversible procedure
5. Loss of bone integrity

Estrogen

Agents include Estradiol Patch, DES®, Estraderm®, Climara®, Stilphostrol®, and Estradurin®

Pros
1. As effective as orchiectomy at achieving castrate-level testosterone
2. Relatively inexpensive compared to other hormonal drugs
3. Requires no surgery

Cons
1. Risk of cardiovascular problems (heart attack, stroke, blood clots)
2. Loss of sexual libido, hot flashes, fluid retention
3. Breast enlargement and/or tenderness
4. Does not supress adrenal androgens

LHRH Agonists

Agents include Lupron®, Zoladex®, TRELSTAR®, and Viadur®.

Pros
1. As effective as orchiectomy, without surgery
2. Low risk of cardiovascular problems
3. Fewer menopausal side effects than estrogen

Cons
1. Expensive ($5000 or more annually)
2. Risk of tumor flare
3. High risk of erectile dysfunction and loss of libido
4. Hot flashes
5. Skin rash and irritation at injection site
6. Does not suppress adrenal androgens
7. Loss of bone integrity

Anti-androgens

Agents Evamist®, Divigel, Minivelle®, Casodex®, Nilandron®, and Androcur®.

Pros
1. Block adrenal androgens
2. Do not require surgery
3. Lower risk of testosterone flare caused by LHRH analogs
4. May increase survival in combination with orchiectomy, or LHRH analogs, or estrogen

Cons
1. Expensive ($5000 or more annually)
2. Diarrhea (less than 10%)
3. Small risk of liver toxicity (requiring monitor)
4. Some risk of breast enlargement and/or tenderness

Hormonal Therapy, DART and Brachytherapy

Points and Counterpoints

Point *(Brachytherapy Extrapolation)*
Hormones plus radiation are at least additive, probably synergistic in enhancing local tumor eradication and affecting subclinical systemic tumor population, especially with high risk patient groups as demonstrated in the following randomized trials:

➤ European Organization for Research and Treatment of Cancer (EORTC) (T_1-T_2 Grade 3, or T_{3-4} – 1 month EBRT alone vs. Goserelin (Zoladex®) during and 3 yrs after)

➤ Radiation Therapy Oncology Group (RTOG) 92-02 (T_{2C}-T_4, EBRT with Goserelin 2 months before and during only vs. 24 months after)

➤ RTOG 85-31 (T_1-T_2N_1, T_3, pathologic T_3, EBRT alone vs. EBRT followed by Goserelin indefinitely)

➤ RTOG 86-10 (large T_2 or T_3-T_4, EBRT alone vs. Flutamide/Goserelin 2 months prior and during

Counterpoint
All randomized trials used conventional EBRT doses (65-70 GY), a lower dose than that delivered by DART and IMRT.

➤ Importance of dose in optimizing bio-chemical outcome for 3D-CRT/IMRT has been established

Zelefsky, J Urol, Vol 166, 2001

➤ Importance of dose in optimizing bio-chemical outcome after brachytherapy has also been established

Stock, IJROBP, Vol 41, 1998
Martinez, IJROBP, Vol 53, 2002
Dattoli, Cancer, Vol 97, 2003

➤ Further evaluation of RTOG trials demonstrates improved 5 year overall survival for patients with Gleason 8-10 who received higher EBRT doses:

Valicenti, J Clin Onc, Vol 18, 2000

➤ In all series reporting biochemical advantage for high risk patients, follow-up of hormone naïve patients has been statistically longer than that of hormonally manipulated patients

➤ 5 year biochemical progression-free survival of 20% reported with Gleason 8-10 with RP alone, 65% RP with adjuvant EBRT supporting an aggressive local-regional approach (vs. sub-clinical systemic approach)
Do, Urology, Vol 57, 2001

Point

➤ ADT has been demonstrated to be the most important prognostic factor for intermediate and high risk patients undergoing mono-therapeutic brachytherapy
Lee, IJROBP, Vol 52, 2002

➤ ADT plus brachytherapy has been shown to improve negative post-implant biopsy result
Stock, Cancer, Vol 89, 2000

Counterpoint

➤ When stratified into low dose vs. high dose (satisfactory vs. unsatisfactory) implants, the above hormone favorable studies are no longer significant
Stock, Cancer, Vol 89, 2000

Point

➤ ADT plus brachytherapy with or without supplemental EBRT has been shown to improve 8-year biochemical outcome in high risk patients.
Merrick, Int J Radiat Oncol Biol Phys, 2005 Jan 1; 61(1):32-43.

APPENDIX A

DECIDING WHAT IS BEST FOR YOU

Consult with your physician, and by all means, obtain second and third opinions whenever possible, preferably from physicians with different specialties. If you have already been to a urologist, it is worthwhile to visit a radiation oncologist or medical oncologist (those with experience with hormones and chemotherapy).

Join a support group such as US TOO!, or PAACT. If you belong to any of the computer on-line services, check out the medical and health bulletin boards and mailing lists for the latest information and announcements for prostate cancer patients. Keep your personal plan of action updated.

What to Remember

- Obtain all of the advice and counsel that you can, but keep in mind that the decisions are ultimately yours to make.

- Be positive—if you have been properly staged and treated, the odds are in your favor on not having a recurrence.

- If you should have a rising PSA over time after initial treatment, don't panic. Get further tests, and if appropriate, get a biopsy, preferably guided by color flow Doppler ultrasound.

- The secret to success with prostate cancer is catching the disease early, and that is also true for recurrence.

- If testing confirms cancer, learn all you can about your options. Get second and third opinions. Become informed and empowered. Become involved with solving your problem. It's your life and body. Go for it!

- Life is full of problems and challenges. Solve this problem like any other big problem:
    1. Identify the problem.
    2. Get all the facts to confirm that you have a problem.
    3. Learn what options are available to you and weigh them carefully.
    4. Choose a qualified doctor who is experienced and with whom you are comfortable.
    5. Initiate and follow through with the solution.
- Don't be afraid to ask for help from your spouse or partner, from your family and your friends. It is more important than ever for you to turn to loved ones to get the emotional and spiritual support you need. This disease can be a difficult struggle for us, but we are not alone, and our mental attitude, prayers and our fighting spirit really can make all the difference.

To be a cancer survivor, you must first be a cancer fighter!

APPENDIX B

GLOSSARY OF MEDICAL TERMS

3D-CRT (3-Dimensional Conformal Radiation Therapy): See Conformal Radiotherapy.

5-alpha reductase (5-AR): an enzyme that converts testosterone to dihydrotestosterone (DHT).

Adenocarcinoma: A cancer originating in glandular tissue. Prostate cancer is classified as adenocarcinoma of the prostate.

Adjuvant: An additional treatment used to increase the effectiveness of the primary therapy. Radiation therapy and hormonal therapy are often used as adjuvant treatments following a radical prostatectomy. Compare Neoadjuvant.

Agonist: A chemical substance that combines with a receptor on a cell and initiates an activity or reaction. See LHRH analogs.

Algorithm: A step-by-step procedure for solving a problem or accomplishing some end, especially by a computer.

Analog: A man-made chemical compound that is structurally similar to one produced naturally by the body. See LHRH analogs.

Anastomotic stricture: narrowing, usually by scarring, of an anastomotic suture line.

Androgen: A hormone that produces male characteristics. See testosterone.

Androgen ablation therapy: A therapy designed to inhibit the body's production of testosterones.

Androgen-dependent cells: Prostate cancer cells which are nourished by male hormones and therefore are capable of being destroyed by hormone deprivation (also known as androgen-sensitive cells).

Androgen-independent cells: Prostate cancer cells which are not dependent on male hormones and therefore do not respond to hormonal therapy (also known as androgen-insensitive cells).

Anesthetic: A drug that produces general or local loss of physical sensations, particularly pain. A "spinal" is the injection of a local anesthetic into the area surrounding the spinal cord.

Aneuploid: Having an abnormal number of chromosomes, as revealed by ploidy analysis. Aneuploid prostate cancer cells tend not to respond well to androgen deprivation therapy (ADT).

Angiogenesis: The body's formation of new blood vessels. Some anti-cancer drugs work by blocking angiogenesis, thus preventing blood from reaching and nourishing a tumor.

Antagonist: A chemical substance in the body that acts to reduce the physiological activity of another chemical substance.

Anti-androgens: Drugs such as Casodex that block the activity of androgens produced by the adrenal glands at the cellular receptor sites. Androgens can block or neutralize the effects of testosterone and DHT on prostate cancer cells.

Antibody: A protein produced by the body that counteracts the toxic effects of a foreign substance, organism, or disease within the body.

Antigen: A foreign substance such as a virus or bacterium that causes an immune response or the formation of an antibody.

Antineoplastic: Inhibits growth and proliferation of cancer cells.

Antioxidants: Any substances which delay the process of oxidation in the body.

Apoptosis: The normal molecular mechanism which governs the life span of cells so that they die in a very organized way. Cancerous cells are resistant to normal apoptosis.

Benign: A non-cancerous condition. See also Benign Prostatic Hypertrophy.

Benign Prostatic Hypertrophy (BPH): Also called Benign Prostatic Hyperplasia, BPH is a non-cancerous condition of the prostate that results in a growth of tumorous tissue and increase in the size of the prostate.

Biopsy: A procedure involving the removal of tissue from the body of the patient. Removed tissue is typically examined microscopically by a pathologist in order to make a precise diagnosis of the patient's condition.

Bone scan: An imaging technique used to detect bone metastases, which appear as "hot spots" on the film. It is far more sensitive than the conventional x-ray.

BPH: See Benign Prostatic Hypertrophy.

Brachytherapy: A form of radiation therapy in which radioactive seeds are implanted into the prostate to deliver radiation directly to the tumor. Also referred to as seed implantation, or seeding.

Cancer: A cellular malignancy typically forming tumors. Unlike benign tumors, these tend to invade surrounding tissues and spread to distant sites of the body.

Carcinoma: A malignant tumor made up chiefly of epithelial cells, or those cells that form the lining of an organ or cavity. See Adenocarcinoma.

Castrate Range: The level of the body's testosterone after orchiectomy (also referred to as castration). This is the range or level, which is used by physicians as a point of comparison for those drugs, which attempt to decrease the testosterone level.

CAT Scan (or CT Scan): See Computer Tomography.

cGy: Abbreviation for centigray; a unit of radiation equivalent to the older unit called a "rad."

Chemotherapy: The treatment of cancer using chemicals that deter the growth of cancer cells.

Collimator: A device that organizes radiation such that only parallel rays or beams emanate.

Combination Hormonal Therapy (CHT): Also referred to as Combined Hormonal Blockade (CHB), or Combined Androgen Deprivation Therapy (ADT). The preferred term is ADT, often designated with a number referring to the number of agents used (i.e., monotherapy ADT, ADT2, ADT3). This combined therapy can utilize a number of mechanisms, including surgical or medical ADT, anti-androgens, 5-alpha reductase inhibitors, estrogenic compounds, agents that block adrenal androgen production, and agents that decrease the receptivity of the androgen receptor.

Combination Therapy: Refers generally to any combination of treatment modalities used to treat prostate cancer.

Computer Tomography: Computer generated cross-sectional images of a portion of the body. Also called CT or CAT scan.

Conformal Radiotherapy: A radiation treatment conforming precisely to the size and shape of the prostate, with the use of computerized planning and state-of-the-art imaging techniques. 3-Dimensional Conformal Radiation Therapy (3D-CRT) utilizes this sophisticated approach to treatment planning, as does the even more advanced Intensity Modulated Radiation Therapy (IMRT).

Cryosurgery (also referred to as Cryotherapy or Cryoablation): The freezing of tissue with the use of liquid nitrogen or Argon gas probes. When used to treat prostate cancer, the cryoprobes are guided by transrectal ultrasound.

Cytokine: Any of a class of immuno-regulatory substances that are secreted by cells of the immune system.

DHT (dihydrotestosterone): The active form of the male hormone, testosterone, produced after testosterone is transformed by an enzyme known as 5-alpha reductase.

Diagnosis: Evaluation of a patient's symptoms and/or test results, with the intent of identifying and verifying the existence of any underlying disease or abnormal condition.

Digital Rectal Examination (DRE): A procedure in which the physician inserts a gloved, lubricated finger into the rectum to examine the prostate gland for signs of cancer.

DNA (Deoxyribonucleic Acid): A complex protein that is the carrier of genetic information that determines the physical development and growth of living organisms.

Doppler Ultrasound Technique: A machine that sends out ultrasonic waves that pick up the velocity of blood flow through the veins and are transmitted as sound to make an image.

Doubling Time: The time it takes for a tumor or cancerous focus to double in size.

Downsizing: The use of hormonal therapy or other forms of intervention to reduce tumor volume prior to primary, curative treatment.

Downstaging: The use of hormonal therapy or other forms of intervention to lower the clinical stage of prostate cancer prior to primary, curative treatment.

Ejaculatory Ducts: The tubular passages through which semen reaches the prostatic urethra during orgasm.

Ejaculation: The release of semen through the penis during orgasm.

Endorectal MRI: Magnetic resonance imaging of the prostate gland using a probe inserted into the rectum. Dynamic Contrast Enhanced MRI is the most effective form of magnetic resonance imaging.

Enzyme: A chemical substance produced by living cells that causes chemical reactions to take place while not being changed itself.

Erectile Dysfunction (also referred to as ED or impotence): The loss of ability to produce and/or sustain an erection sufficient for intercourse.

Estrogen: A female sex hormone that can be used as a form of therapy to inhibit the production of testosterone in patients diagnosed with prostate. cancer.

External Beam Radiation Therapy (EBRT): A form of radiation therapy that utilizes radiation delivered by an external source (machine) and directed at a target area to be radiated. In contrast to EBRT, brachytherapy utilizes radiation sources (seeds) that are internal, implanted in the target tissue. EBRT may use conventional photons, protons, neutrons or electrons.

Extracapsular Extension: Used to describe prostate cancer that has spread outside the prostate gland.

False Negative: An erroneous negative test result. For example, an imaging test that fails to show the presence of a cancer tumor later found by biopsy to be present in the patient is said to have returned a false negative result.

False Positive: A positive test result that mistakenly identifies a state or condition that does not in fact exist.

Feraheme (Ferumoxytol): A ferromagnetic nanoparticle which is taken up by normal macrophages with the lymph nodes.

Fistula: With regard to prostate cancer, an abnormal passage due to injury or disease that connects an abscess or hollow organ to the surface of the body or to another hollow organ. If there is significant damage to the rectal wall proximate to the bladder, a fistula may occur between the bladder and rectum.

Flare Reaction: A testosterone surge caused by the initial use of an LHRH analog, causing a temporary increase of tumor growth and symptoms (known as clinical flare), or an increase in PSA (biochemical flare).

Foley Catheter: A catheter inserted in the penis and threaded through the urethra to the bladder where it is held in place with a tiny, inflated balloon. It removes urine from the bladder and can be used to irrigate the urethra and prevent blood clots.

Free PSA: PSA that is unattached to any major protein in the blood. Free PSA is associated with benign prostate growth. The percentage of free PSA is derived by dividing the free-PSA level by the total-PSA x 100. Studies have show that men with free PSA % > 25% were at low risk for prostate cancer, while men with PSA % < 10% were at high risk for having prostate cancer.

Frozen Section: A technique in which removed tissue is frozen, cut into thin slices, and stained for microscopic examination. A pathologist can rapidly complete a frozen section analysis, and for this reason, it is commonly used during surgery to quickly provide the surgeon with vital information.

Gland: An aggregation of cells (a structure or organ) that secretes a substance for use or discharge from the body.

Gland Volume: The size in cubic centimeters (cc) or grams of the prostate gland.

Gleason Score: A widely used method for classifying the cellular differentiation of cancerous tissue. The less the cancerous cells appear like normal cells, the more malignant the cancer. Two grades of 1-5, identifying the two most common degrees of differentiation present in the examined tissue sample, are added together to produce the Gleason score. High numbers indicate greater differentiation and more aggressive cancer. The grading system is named after its originator, Donald Gleason, M.D.

Globulin: Any of a number of simple proteins that occur widely in plant and animal tissues.

Gynecomastia: A side effect involving breast enlargement and tenderness, associated with various hormonal therapies that increase the level of estrogens in the body.

HDR brachytherapy: High Dose Rate brachytherapy involves the temporary insertion of radioactive iridium isotopes into the prostate gland using transrectal ultrasound guidance.

Hematuria: Blood in the urine.

Hereditary: Inherited genetically from parents and earlier generations.

Holistic Medicine: Medical care, which considers the patient as a whole, including his or her physical, mental, emotional, spiritual, social and economic needs.

Hormone: A substance produced by one tissue or gland and transported by the bloodstream to another to effect or regulate physiological activity such as metabolism and growth.

Hormonal therapy: Cancer treatment involving the blockage of hormone production by surgical or chemical means. Because prostate cancer is usually dependent on male hormones to grow, hormonal therapy can be an effective means of alleviating symptoms and retarding the development of the disease.

Hormone refractory prostate cancer: Prostate cancer that is androgen independent, and therefore, unresponsive to hormonal therapies.

Hot Flash: A side effect of some forms of hormonal therapy, experienced as a sudden rush of warmth to the face, neck, and upper body.

Imaging: Radiology techniques that are often computer-enhanced and allow the physician to visualize areas inside the body that would not normally be visible.

Impotence: See Erectile Dysfunction.

Incontinence: A loss of urinary control.

There are various kinds and degrees of incontinence. Overflow incontinence is a condition in which the bladder retains urine after voiding. As a consequence, the bladder remains full most of the time, resulting in involuntary seepage of urine from the bladder. Stress incontinence is the involuntary discharge of urine when there is increased pressure upon the bladder, as in coughing or straining to lift heavy objects. Total incontinence is the failure of ability to voluntarily exercise control over the sphincters of the bladder neck and urethra, resulting in total loss of retentive ability.

Inflammation: Redness or swelling caused by injury or infection.

Informed Consent: Permission to proceed given by a patient after being fully informed of the purposes and potential consequences of a medical procedure.

Intensity Modulated Radiation Therapy (IMRT): The most recent state-of-the-art, computer-aided technique for delivering higher doses of radiation more accurately than either conventional External Beam Radiation or Conformal Radiation. The most advanced form of IMRT is Dynamic Adaptive Radiotherapy (DART).

Intermittent Androgen Deprivation (IAD): A temporary discontinuation of hormonal therapy that allows for a return to natural testosterone production in order to spare the patient from symptoms associated with androgen deprivation. Also referred to as Intermittent Hormonal Therapy (IHT).

Intravenous Pyelogram (IVP): A test that utilizes the injection of a special dye to check for injury or the spread of cancer to the kidneys and bladder.

Investigational: A drug or procedure allowed by the FDA for use in clinical trails, but not necessarily reimbursed.

Isodose Line: A line or two-dimensional shape that circumscribes an area receiving a radiation dose greater than or equal to a specified amount.

Laparoscopic Lymphadenectomy: The removal of pelvic lymph nodes with a laparoscope via four small incisions in the lower abdomen.

LH (Luteinizing Hormone): A chemical signal originating in the pituitary gland that causes the testes to make testosterone.

LHRH Analogs (or LHRH Agonists): Synthetic compounds that are chemically similar to Luteinizing Hormone Releasing Hormone (LHRH), used to suppress testicular production of testosterone. The most commonly prescribed LHRH analogs are Lupron® and Zoldex® Eligard® and Trelstar®. See also Luteinizing Hormone-Releasing Hormone (LHRH).

LHRH Antagonist: A chemical agent that blocks the LHRH receptor without the testosterone surge associated with

LHRH analogs. LHRH antagonists include Abarelix (Plenaxis®).

Linear Accelerator: A high energy x-ray machine generating radiation fields for external beam radiation therapy. These machines are typically mounted with a collimator (or multileaf collimator) in a gantry that rotates vertically around the patient being treated.

Localized Prostate Cancer: Cancer that is confined to the prostate gland, and therefore, considered curable.

Luteinizing Hormone-Releasing Hormone (LHRH): A chemical signal originating in the hypothalamus that causes the pituitary to make LH, which in turn stimulates the testicles to make testosterone.

Lymphadenectomy: The removal and examination of lymph nodes to precisely diagnose and stage cancer. See also Laparascopic Lymphadenectomy.

Lymph Node: A small, bean-shaped mass of tissue located throughout the body along the vessels of the lymphatic system. The lymph nodes filter out bacteria and other toxins, as well as cancer cells.

Magnetic Resonance Imaging (MRI): A painless, non-invasive technique using strong magnetic fields to produce detailed images of internal body structures. An MRI scan usually takes about 45 minutes per site.

Malignancy: A tumorous growth of cancer cells.

Malignant: Having the invasive and metastatic properties of cancer. Tending to become progressively worse and to result in death.

Margin: See Surgical Margin.

Metalloprotease Inhibitors: Drugs used to suppress the body's production of certain enzymes.

Metastasis: The spread of cancer, by way of the blood stream or lymphatic system, beyond the boundaries of the organ or structure where the cancer originated. Metastases is the plural. Metastatic refers to the characteristics associated with cancer that has spread or a secondary tumor.

Metastatic Work-Up: A group of tests, including bone scans, x-rays, and blood tests, to ascertain whether cancer has metastasized.

Monoclonal Antibody (mAb): An antibody that is directed against one specific protein (antigen).

Morbidity: Unhealthy consequences and complications resulting from treatment.

MRI: See Magnetic Resonance Imaging.

Nadir: The lowest point. Doctors sometimes use this as a verb to describe return of cancer or treatment failure. The PSA nadir refers to a minimum PSA value that should be maintained after treatment if the cancer has been successfully eradicated.

Necrosis: Death of cells or tissues caused by disease or injury.

Neoadjuvant: The use of a different type of therapy before primary, curative treatment. For example, neoadjuvant Androgen Deprivation Therapy is often used prior to radiation therapy or radical surgery, with the intent of improving the effectiveness of the primary treatment by reducing the size of the tumor and/or prostate gland.

Nerve-sparing: A procedure used during radical prostatectomy in which the surgeon attempts to save the nerves (neurovascular bundles) that allow for normal sexual functions.

Neurovascular Bundles: Strands of interwoven nerves and veins that run down the side of the prostate. The bundles contain microscopic nerves that are essential for erection; they also contain arteries and veins. Cutting the nerves in the bundles during surgery, or otherwise harming them in another procedure, usually renders the patient impotent.

Nocturia: Getting up at night to urinate.

Non-invasive: Not involving any incision in the body.

Oncogenes: Genes associated with tumor growth.

Oncology: The branch of medical science dealing with tumors. A medical oncologist is a specialist in the study of cancerous tumors.

Organ-confined Disease (OCD): Prostate cancer that is confined to the prostate capsule, as indicated clinically or pathologically.

Orchiectomy: A simple operation that involves surgical removal of the testicles, which produce most of the body's testosterone.

Osteoporosis: A decrease in bone mass and density causing fragility and porosity.

Overstaging: An assessment of an overly high clinical stage at initial diagnosis.

Palliative: Affording symptomatic pain relieve but not cure or remission.

Palpable: Capable of being felt when examined by touch or manipulation.

PAP: See Prostatic Acid Phosphatase.

Pathologist: A doctor who specializes in the examination of cells and tissues removed from the body.

PBRT: See Proton Beam Radiation Therapy.

Perineum: The area of the body between the anus and scrotum. A perineal procedure uses this area as the point of entry into the body.

Perineural Invasion: Describing cancer, which has spread from the prostate to the nerve bundles.

Periprostatic: Relating to the soft tissues immediately proximate to the prostate gland.

Photon: The quantum of electromagnetic energy, described as having zero mass and no electric charge. X-rays are high energy photons.

Placebo: A sugar pill often taken by participants in a medical study. Patients taking a placebo are compared to patients taking actual medications.

Ploidy Analysis: A pathological analysis to determine the number of sets of chromosomes in a cell.

Proctitis: Inflammation of the rectum.

Prognosis: A forecast of the course of a disease and future prospects of the patient.

Progression: A change in the status of the cancer indicating the condition has progressed and worsened.

Pro-oxidant: A term to describe substances that aid in oxidation.

ProstaScint® Scan: An imaging technique sometimes used determine whether or not cancer has spread to distant sites by using monoclonal antibodies.

Prostate Capsule: The outer membranous covering of the prostate gland.

Prostatectomy: The surgical removal of part or all of the prostate gland.

Prostate Specific Antigen (PSA): A blood test that measures a substance manufactured solely by prostate gland cells. An elevated reading indicates an abnormal condition of the prostate gland, either benign or malignant. It is presently the most sensitive tumor marker for the identification and monitoring of prostate cancer.

Prostatic Acid Phosphatase (PAP): An enzyme produced by the prostate that is elevated (3.0 or higher) in many patients when prostate cancer has spread beyond the prostate.

Prostatitis: An infection or inflammation of the prostate gland that is treatable with medications.

Proton Beam Radiation Therapy (PBRT): A form of radiation therapy that utilizes protons as the source of energy (as opposed to X-rays or neutrons).

PSA: See Prostate Specific Antigen.

PSA Bounce (or PSA Bump): A rise in PSA level after first having a reduction in PSA after radiation therapy.

PSA Nadir: The lowest PSA value after a particular treatment.

PSA Velocity (PSAV): The rate of increase of the PSA level, expressed as nanograms per milliliter per year.

Radiation Therapy (RT): The use of high energy rays to kill cancer cells and malignant tissue.

Radiation Urethritis: Inflammation of the urethra caused by radiation therapy.

Radical Prostatectomy: An operation to remove the entire prostate gland and seminal vesicles.

Radiosensitivity: The degree to which a type of cancer responds to radiation therapy.

RBA or Relative Biological Effectiveness: A scale used to compare the intensity of radiation associated with various atomic particles.

Receptor: A cellular docking site that interacts with a specific protein or enzyme (called a ligand). The interaction typically leads to the synthesis of other substances such as proteins, hormones or enzymes.

Recurrence: Return of the cancer following remission or treatment intended as curative. Local recurrence indicates a return of the cancer at the site of origin. Distant recurrence indicates the appearance of one or more metastases of the disease.

Refractory: A term indicating that the cancer no longer responds to the current therapy.

Remission: Complete or partial disappearance of the signs and symptoms of the disease. The period during which a disease remains under control, without progressing. Even complete remission does not necessarily indicate cure.

Resection: The surgical removal of a part of an organ or structure.

Risk: The probability that a particular even will or will not happen.

RP: See Radical Prostatectomy.

RT: See Radiation Therapy.

Rx: The standard abbreviation for prescription.

Salvage Treatment: A medical term for "Plan B." It means a patient must undergo another form of treatment because the first therapy was not successful. Salvage therapy may incur a higher rate of side effects.

Saw Palmetto: A nutrient extracted from the saw palmetto shrub, which is considered by some to aid the body's immune system.

Seed Implantation (SI): A minimally invasive procedure by which radioactive seeds are implanted into the prostate gland to destroy cancer. Also referred to as seeding and brachytherapy.

Selenium: A non-metallic element thought to be beneficial as a nutrient; it is often included in multivitamin supplements.

Seminal Vesicles: Glands that, like the prostate, support male reproduction. Fluid secreted by these glands regulates the consistency of semen.

Side Effect: A reaction to a treatment or medication, usually referring to an undesirable effect.

Sphincter: A circular muscle which contracts to close an orifice. The urethral sphincter squeezes the urethra shut, providing urinary control.

Staging: The testing process by which the extent and severity of a known cancer is evaluated according to an established system of classification. It is used to help determine appropriate therapy. See TNM Staging and Whitmore-Jewett Staging.

Surgical Margin: The outer edge of the tissue removed during a radical prostatectomy. The surgical margin may be "negative," indicating that no cancer is present and a better prognosis, or "positive," indicating that not all of the cancer has been removed.

Systemic: Throughout the body and affecting the entire body.

T-Cell: An immune system cell or lymphocyte that directs an immune response to malignant or infected cells.

Testes: Two male reproductive glands located inside the scrotum. The testes are the primary sources for testosterone. Also called testicles.

Testosterone: A male sex hormone chiefly produced by the testicles.

Thrombotic: Causing or relating to blood clotting.

TNM Staging: The most widely used classification system for evaluating the extent of prostate cancer. TNM refers to tumor, nodes and metastases. See Staging.

Transrectal: Through the rectum.

Transurethral: Through the urethra.

Transrectal Ultrasonography: See Ultrasound.

Transurethral Resection of the Prostate (TURP): A surgical procedure to remove tissue obstructing the urethra. The technique involves the insertion of an instrument called a resectoscope into the penile urethra, and is intended to relieve obstruction of urine flow due to enlargement of the prostate.

Tumor: An excessive growth of cells that is caused by uncontrolled and disorderly cell replacement. Abnormal tissue growth may be benign or malignant. See also Benign, Malignant.

TURP: See Transurethral Resection of the Prostate.

Ultrasound (Transrectal Ultrasonography): A painless, non-invasive diagnostic imaging technique using sound waves to create an echo pattern that reveals the structure of organs and tissues. It does not use x-rays.

Understaging: An overly low assessment of clinical stage at diagnosis.

Urethra: The tube that carries urine from the bladder and semen from the prostate out of the body through the penis.

Urologist: A physician who specializes in the diagnosis and the medical and surgical treatment of problems in the urinary and male reproductive systems.

USPIO: This technology uses ultrasmall superparamagnetic iron oxide (USPIO) as an MRI contrast agent for the identification of cancer metastasis in lymph nodes.

Vasectomy: A surgical procedure to render a man sterile by cutting the vas deferens, thus eliminating the passage of sperm from the testes to the prostate.

Vasoactive: Causing the dilation or constriction of blood vessels.

Vesicle: A small sac containing fluid, as in seminal vesicles.

Whitmore-Jewett Staging: A classification system for evaluating the extent of prostate cancer. This system is less widely used for the designation of stage than is TNM staging.

X-rays: High energy radiation that can be used at low levels of intensity to make images of the body's internal structures, or at high intensity for radiation therapy.

APPENDIX C

THE WARNING SIGNS OF PROSTATE CANCER

There are often no warning signs of prostate cancer. In some cases the following symptoms may indicate the presence of the disease. However, please be aware that these symptoms may also be due to benign conditions of the prostate, or other conditions entirely unrelated to prostate cancer:

- ✔ Elevated or rising PSA
- ✔ Abnormal Digital Rectal Exam
- ✔ Blood in urine
- ✔ Pain or difficulty urinating
- ✔ Increased urge to urinate, especially at night
- ✔ Hesitant or intermittent urinary flow
- ✔ Pain or discomfort in area of prostate
- ✔ Unusual and unexplained weight loss
- ✔ Continual pain in lower back, hips or pelvis
- ✔ Increased voiding urgency
- ✔ Inability to urinate
- ✔ Trouble having or keeping an erection (erectile dysfunction)
- ✔ Weakness or numbness in the legs or feet

ABOUT THE AUTHOR

Michael J. Dattoli, MD

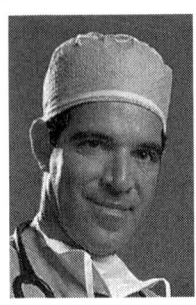

Michael J. Dattoli, MD, is a board-certified radiation oncologist with well over two decades of brachytherapy experience and has performed thousands of prostate implant procedures. He is considered the foremost pioneer in the field, optimizing brachytherapy designs to maximize tumor eradication and minimize symptoms. He has also been the leading trailblazer in the development of Dynamic Adaptive Radiotherapy (DART), utilizing all of the state-of-the-art modalities associated with 4-Dimensional Image-Guided Intensity Modulated Radiotherapy (3D-IMRT). Dr. Dattoli has successfully applied the same technologies to other forms of cancer, including breast, head and neck, GI, GYN, sarcomas and lung malignancies. He is a noted author and speaker in this complex field of medicine.

Dr. Dattoli attended the University of California at Berkeley and was the Valedictorian of his class at Vassar College; he earned his medical degree at Mount Sinai School of Medicine, Radiation Oncology at New York University Medical Center, then distinguished himself at Memorial Sloan-Kettering Cancer Center and New York Hospital-Cornell University Medical Center, as the Special Fellow in Brachytherapy. He was appointed Associate Professor in Brachytherapy and Radiation Oncology at Memorial Sloan- Kettering Cancer Center in New York and at New York Hospital-Cornell University Medical Center prior to relocating to Florida.

Dr. Dattoli also serves on multiple journal editorial review boards. Government appointments include "The Prostate Cancer Task Force" in Florida and consultant to the "Washington Oncology Roundtable Advisory Committee". He was selected by the International Association of Oncologists as a Leading Physician of the World and top Brachytherapist.

THE DATTOLI CANCER FOUNDATION MISSION

The Dattoli Cancer Foundation, sponsor of the Prostate Cancer Resource Network, is a 501(c)(3), tax-exempt charitable organization, whose mission is

- to raise awareness of the wide-spread incidence of Prostate Cancer and the need for early and annual screenings;

- to provide information and support to men newly diagnosed with Prostate Cancer as well as to those with recurrent Prostate Cancer, and

- to foster research into better diagnostic tools and treatment options for Prostate Cancer.

Gifts to the Dattoli Foundation make possible publications like this one, and are welcomed anytime. A copy of the official registration and financial information may be obtained from the Division of Consumer Services by calling toll-free (800-435-7352) within the state. Registration does not imply endorsement, approval or recommendations by the state.

Dattoli Cancer Foundation
2803 Fruitville Road
Sarasota, FL 34237
941/365-5599
800/915-1001
fax: 941/332-2317
www.dattolifoundation.org

ORDER MORE BOOKLETS IN THE SERIES

This *Prostate Cancer Essentials for Survival* booklet was prepared and distributed by the Dattoli Cancer Foundation, which is dedicated to providing information, hope and encouragement to prostate cancer patients and their loved ones. Additional booklets in this series are planned for publication in the near future. Previous titles include:

- ✓ *IMRT with DART and Brachytherapy*
- ✓ *Dynamic Adaptive Radiation Therapy: A Primer on DART, the Most Comprehensive Solution for Informed Patients*
- ✓ *The Dattoli Challenge: Evaluating Your Prostate Cancer Treatment Options*
- ✓ *Interpreting Your PSA: And Related Prostate Cancer Blood Tests*
- ✓ *Prostate Cancer Recurrence: Need You Be Concerned?*
- ✓ *Prostate Biopsy: When, Why And What To Expect*
- ✓ *Dosimetry and Prostate Cancer Radiotherapy: Precision Design for IMRT and Brachytherapy*

To find out when additional booklets will be released or to order copies of currently available booklets, please contact the Dattoli Cancer Foundation at (800) 915-1001.

Printed in Poland
by Amazon Fulfillment
Poland Sp. z o.o., Wrocław